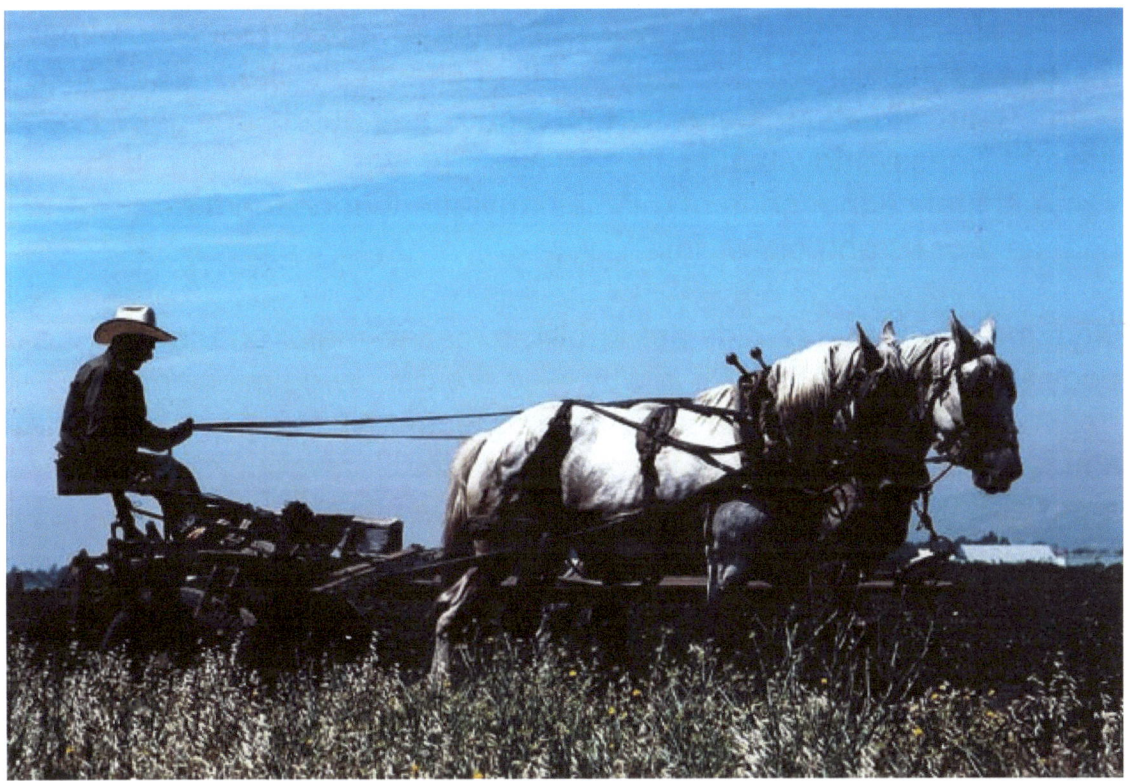

What ever happened to the days of natural food and natural farming?

That is the first question one must begin to answer before one can even begin to look at the facts about our present food chain system.

Sure, the example in the picture above is part of the progress that has come about over the decades. Gone are the days of horse drawn plows. Simply put, we have machines that now do the job like tractors and combines. That type of progress has been good. However, some of the other progress has come with a price tag that is far often too high when it comes to our safety and the safety of our natural resources.

In those same old days, a Farmer simply planted his crops and allowed nature to take it course. Today, we pump hundreds of gallons of water onto those fields, pre-fertilize the ground with chemicals that not only promote growth, which is fine, as well as chemicals to kill off weeds and bugs, many of whose labels all warn not for human consumption, can cause cancer, and are poisons in their own right. At the same time, those who produce these compounds and make money on them all try to claim none of it gets into our food supply. The Beef and Chicken Industry forces the Farmers out there to pump the cows and chickens and pigs all full of chemicals like steroids to promote growth at a faster rate, anti-biotic compounds designed to prevent illness, and vitamins to also aid in growth and claims in the same sentence that none of this has any effect upon the food we consume or us and our children.

Give me a break! Steroids are known to cause major changes in the body structure of people. It is why they are out lawed in Sports to begin with. It was also the carrier in that recent NECC drug case. They cause fertility problems. They cause abnormal growth. They cause heart and digestive illnesses. In addition, we are supposed to buy into the line that none of this in our food is unhealthy.

We now have viruses immune to many anti-biotic compounds showing up more and more. Vitamins in and of themselves occur naturally. So the question becomes do we really need all the extra ones in our food chain to begin with?

When you buy beef at your local store, all of the above is what you are getting.

THE TROUBLE WITH OUR FOOD AND DRUG SUPPLY SYSTEM

By: Paul Karl Hoiland

Author of several different books on subjects ranging from the Council of Foreign Relations, to UFO's, Remote Viewing, Wicca, Warp Drive, and Modern Cosmology now tackles a far more immediate problem when it comes to the health and future of mankind, asking the Big Questions and answering them with who is behind all this and what is the risk to everyone. If you are like most American's getting your meals from the major store chains, don't take another bite till you get the facts, Before you are done you will know the who, what, and why and you will see how this problem spills over into the drug industry also.

You will discover how this once great agricultural nation got suckered into trusting the Big Corporations to both monitor and control every facet of our food supply chain, how those same Corporations managed over time to even control the Federal Agency in charge of protecting the American People and how little you really know what is in that meal before you on the table. You will see how a similar manipulation over time has managed to put the drug companies out there in power over that same Federal Agency.

This is the story of Global Corporate take over of the American Farm from what they grow, to the very chemicals they treat our soil with, on down to the chemicals we ingest in our food everyday being sold to an American public that has become "Lab Rats" in the worldwide control of everything in our lives. They complain about the soda we drink and never say a word about the effects all those chemicals have upon the human body.

Email: joatp2000@yahoo.com

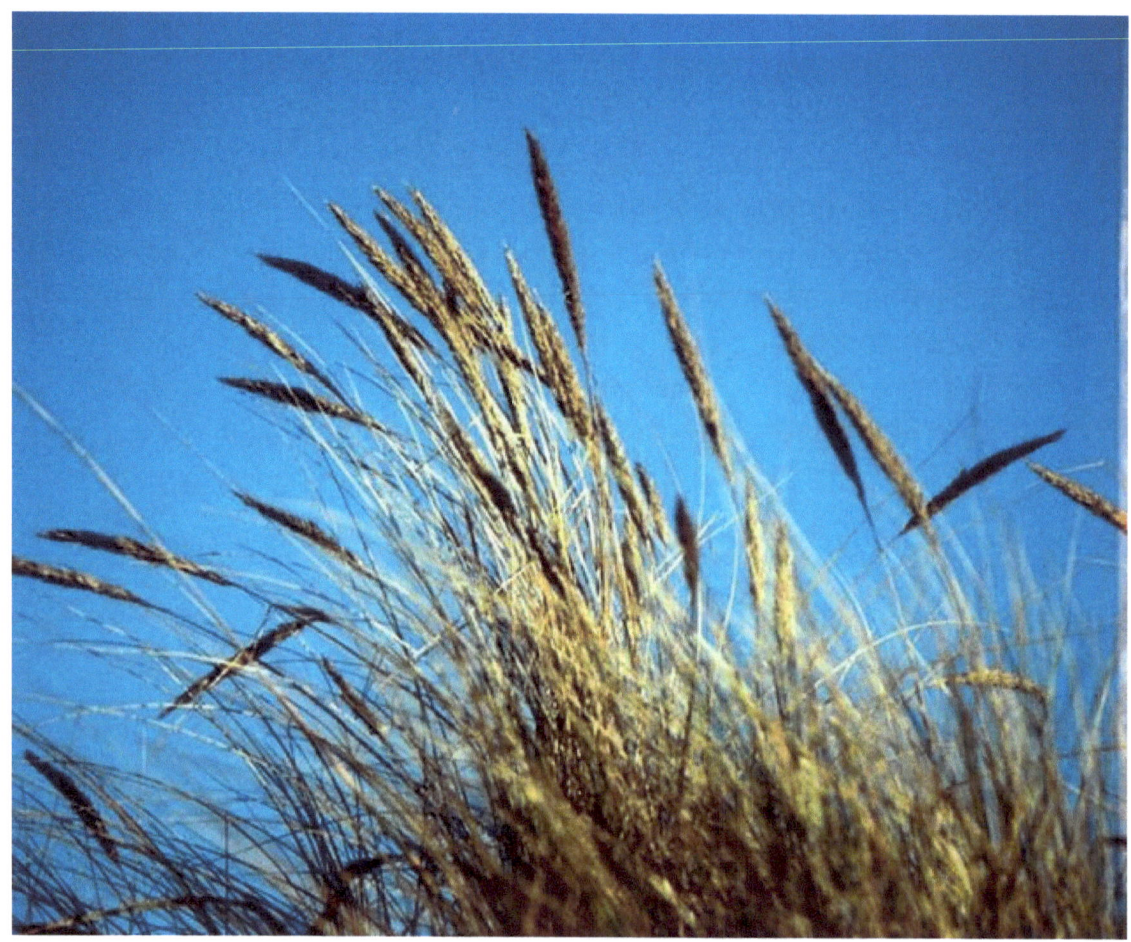

INTRODUCTION

Every time one picks up the Paper, turns on the TV news or reads an article on the Net we see more and more indication of a major problem when it comes to our Food Supply chain and to the Drugs, our Doctors prescribe for us. Just recently, we have the major case of meningitis spread via a Compounding Company in New England, the same company that back in 03 settled a lawsuit out of court on a death due to the same illness being transmitted by the same basic drug. Same company with workers and management that stood around seeing decay and mold on the walls and did nothing. All this under what is supposed to be the watchful eye of our Big Brother Government in the FDA. We now have the beginning of illnesses that at one time where nearly unheard of related to what is in our food and drinking water. We have evidence our youth are developing sexually far earlier than normal, with a strong connection to the drugs and chemicals we put into our food supply all in the name of more profit and progress.

However, very few people bother to look up the facts themselves. They trust our Government to protect them, Companies like Monsanto to make sure our food is safe, and all the while, they keep buying the junk out there being sold in our stores as food. At the same time, these authorities, in control of our food supply chain, manipulate the markets through their interest, dictating those markets and what will be grown where, all in the name of more profit.

Gone are the days of natural corn and grain feed beef. Gone are the days of natural grown chicken, or pork, or even apples. Everything from Corn to beef has chemicals added into them. Stuff like growth hormones, anti-biotics, food coloring, preservatives just to name a few. All stuff virtually untested as far as long-term effects on the human bodies; untested as far as effects on the nature and safety of our food we eat. Then you have a drug industry that spends far more money on development of what amounts to band-aids for the pain many suffer instead of a cure. I know on that last point since my Wife suffers from fibermioalgia, with no solution except painkillers to even begin to function most days.

We have Politicians in this Country that do not have a clue, who like the FDA are bought and sold to the highest bidder, usually the same companies they are supposed to protect us from. These same Agencies literally are in bed with Companies like Monsanto and NECC, to name a few, that have brought so much death and pain to literally hundreds of America citizens.

Unfounded claim, you say. Not really when you begin to look at the facts, when you begin to follow the money trail, when you begin to understand the control the Industry that is supposed to be regulated by the FDA has over the FDA itself and over those who grow and produce our food and our drugs.

This is where Corporate America has brought us and the rest of the World to in its lust for power and more money. To a Nation where it is citizens, with the right to the pursuit of **Life**, **Liberty**, and **Happiness**, has become the lab rats for Big Business. We hear the result of those "Lab Rat" experiments everyday in the News, we see those results in many of our families across the Nation all in the name of Power and Money while our Government stands by, lines their pockets for the next election cycle, and the Agencies in charge turn a blind eye to reality.

We have a country with far too many over weight people, we have a country where diabetic conditions effect many, all the result of the food we consume everyday. At the same time we have ad agencies that promote the ultra thin look and those same food choices that promote an over weight condition. The result is a tread mill run of people with emotional problems when it comes to their image, caught between the idea of the thin and foods far too unfit for consumption that promote an over weight unhealthy condition.

Simply put information is power. The purpose of this book is to arm my fellow American's and human beings with that information compiled together so as to be more informed on the truth and able to make a stand to protect themselves and possible begin to police the Industry out there via how they buy and what they buy and what they do have as choices. An educated citizen is the real protection of democracy when you boil it all down. Educated citizens aware of what is going on tend to vote in ways that are more educated. In the end run, not all the money of those Big Corporations out there buys the votes at the polls, nor does it actually determine what is bought in our food store chains across this country. Take away the power they have in the form of money and you take away all their power and take back this country for its people.

BEEF ITS WHATS FOR DINNER

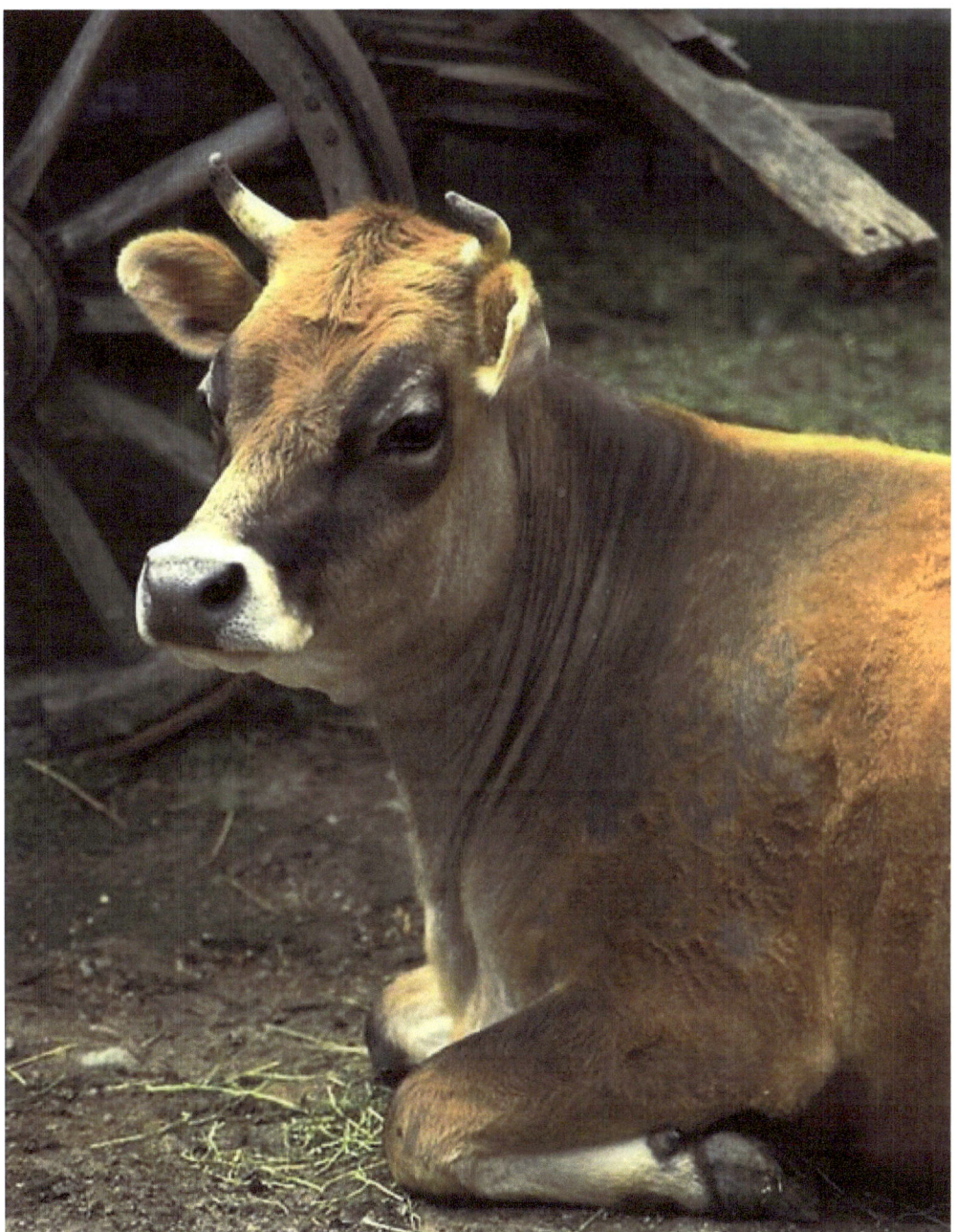

If truth was in our product labeling for real, Beef is what's for diner or 100% grade A beef would be replaced with 95% beef and the rest chemicals. The same goes for our Chicken, our Turkey, our Pigs, and just about everything else we humans consume as food.

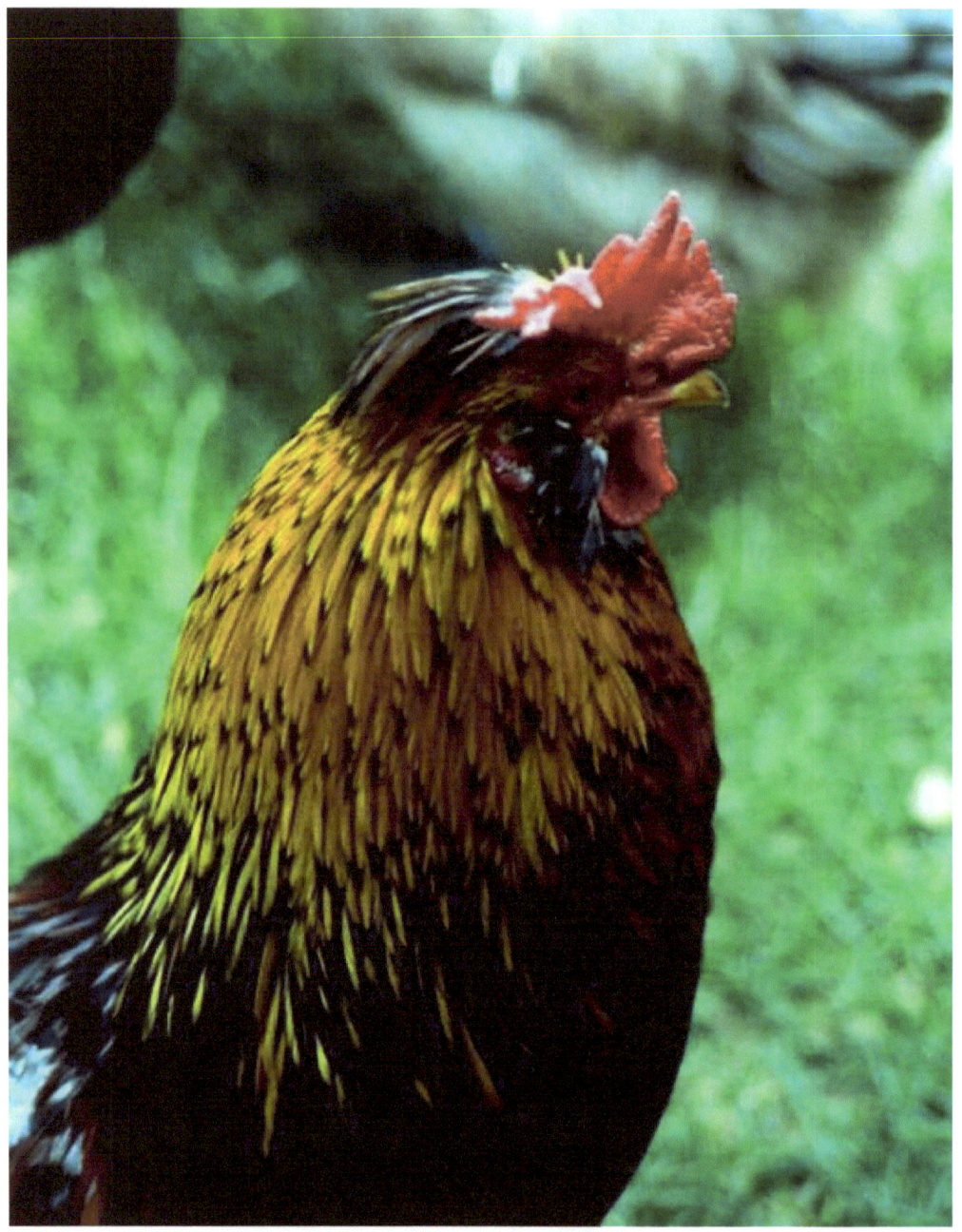

It is all in there to get more pounds out of the products, to grow the product faster so that these Big Companies can all make more profit in the end run. The Chicken you have on a Sunday afternoon got to you faster and with more meat, all because of these same chemicals designed to speed up growth that results in harm to our human bodies. Personally, I would rather have my food on the table take a bit longer to get to market and be safer. If I wanted to ingest these chemicals I would buy them to eat at a local chemical store instead of food from a food store like Kroger, or meat from Tyson, just to name a few. The question we all need to be asking is do we want that chicken above on our table or something that looks like chicken full of chemicals that might have well come out of an oil rig like the one illustrated below. Which for a reason is shown right next to a Farmer's barn and grain silo?

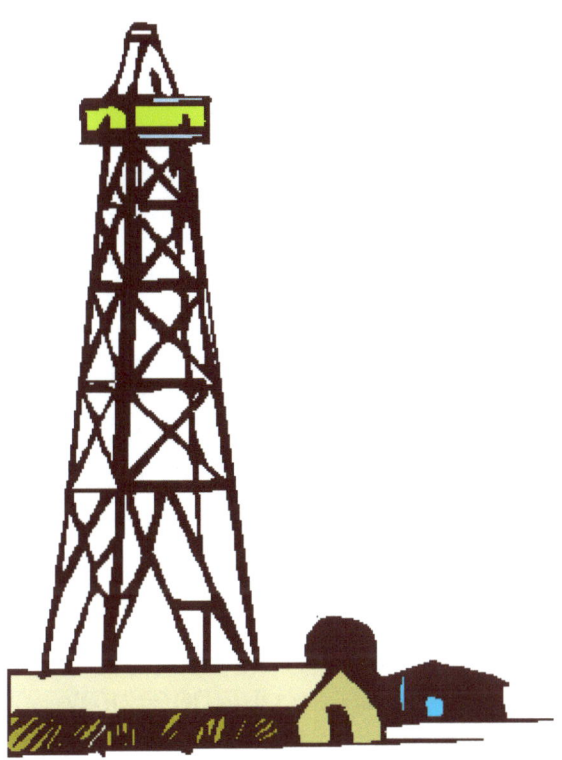

If that picture was, complete it should have included one of those chemical companies on the same property that supplies all the pesticides and herbicides used on our crops and on the hay, we feed our cattle. Basically, boil it all down and that is exactly what we now get at the market they sell us as food. All brought to your diner table via the World Wide Giant Corporations out there like Monsanto and Tyson, all under the so-called watchful eye of the FDA here in America controlled by a Government that long ago lost all pretense of protecting its citizens no matter the Party they belong too. Makes one really take a second look at that nice steak on the grill and think hard about the so-called Conservative Motto about less Government regulations. Seems to me when it comes to our food and drugs we need better regulations, more proper testing, and harsher enforcement of the rules to begin with. Can you really honestly trust either the Government or the Corporations to do the right thing is the first question we should be asking?

When the human race was a Hunter/gather society as a whole, our worst problem was trying to hunt better and gather better. We as a race had to use our minds to think how to do both better. However, that is also, where the whole progress thing that led to our present situation first got started. Along the way from there to here, the thirst for progress changed rational thinking with some wisdom mixed in to pure greed. It may be true as myth paints that Adam was cursed to work hard to get anything out of the soil, out of nature. However, do we have to add in further curses in the form of chemicals all in the name of progress is a completely different subject? That is the subject of what happened to our food chain.

I'd like to say it all began out on the Farm. However, it actually all began in some Corporate Board Room would be more accurate. Basically, the Farmers had a need to grow improved crops to supply the needs of a growing population. In some corporate office, which supplied the needed fertilizer to allow for bigger better crops somebody, proposed finding a way to improve those crops, to make them more resistant to the perils of nature, to genetically alter those plants to achieve a better harvest, to make the cattle out there grow faster and have more beef on them, etc.   Not all of this in and of itself is a bad idea. However, what mutated a decent idea into a monster that took on a life of its own were the dollar signs in the eyes of those corporate officers in that think tank to begin with.

Sure, there are many Corporations involved, not just one. The Chemical Companies, the Big Food Produce Companies, the soda production companies, the sugar companies, just to name a few are all involved in this. One could also add in the fast food outfits in America, who until forced to change their image did little positive towards the average American diet. Even today, though they boast of less fat meals they offer, the actual chemicals in those foods has little changed at all. The fit and trim meals they now offer along side of the older traditional burgers and fry's has less fat, but all the same chemical additives, making what they offer just seem better for you.

Enter Monsanto, started in 1902 and by 1920 had begun to dominate the chemical industry for both industrial and agricultural usage. It has a decade's long history of problems ranging from those with DDT to Agent Orange, to chemical dumping, etc. It dominates the whole farming world with genetically modified seeds and a host of chemicals to utilize in farming for weed control, etc. They spend around 2 million per day in research on genetically modified seeds ranging from corn to wheat. There have been many proven instances of anybody going outside of them being bullied into using their seeds and chemicals alone.

The whole agent orange affair is well documented and the Company has been shown to have known well ahead of time the effects dioxin, Agent Orange's main chemical, had on human bodies long before they sold it to the Government. The result of it's wide spread use by the Government during the Vietnam war is also well documented and resulted in a major lawsuit against the Company.

The Company has a long published history of caring little about the health of the public and far more about the bottom line of profits. In almost every case that has come forward the Company has been shown to have known ahead of time problems with its chemicals via their own internal documents.

One of their biggest tricks for more profit is to insist that Farmers planting their Round Up ready seeds do not save them from year to year, as farmers used to traditionally. This makes for more sales since the Farmers have to buy new seed every year and it gives them virtual control over the Market since Round Up is now the most common used weed control agent in Farming having seeds that can grow even when Round Up is used is almost a must anymore.

The main active agent in Round Up is a well-known Cancer causing chemical Glyphosate. This is just the tip of a much bigger ice burg when it comes to this company. One simply has to look at the long list of chemicals this Company developed to discover the trend they have. DDT, Agent Orange, Round Up, just to name a few.

The most known and proven effect of Genetic modification of seeds is an allergic reaction some people have to these foods. As for the Chemicals used on the plants in the field all are known to pose health problems and yet, little study to see how much of them makes it into the food chain has been done to date. One study actually used a chemical gene that was known to cause problems in butterflies in an attempt to see if it could effect other populations with a noted positive result that is however flawed because of the actual gene involved in the first place, that has never been used in any food supply chain.

There has been questions about these gene modifications making into via cross polonization into say the weed population, however to date no solid evidence of such has come forward. This is an area in need of far more study and the long-term effects of such gene modification on the human body after consumption needs further looked at.

Monsanto brought us NutraSweet. They also exert a huge amount of influence in Washington D.C., which prevents any large-scale meaningful debate. Therefore, while they present themselves as a "life science" or biotechnology firm, they are really a chemical firm and nothing more since their founding.

Take the following as a small example:

- Their attempt to market its genetically engineered products as organic in the United States came under criticism and was fought back -- for now.
- However, that did not stop them trying it in India, using an Indian seed company that they bought in order to use the term "Organic" as a Trojan Horse to enter the huge Indian market, amidst huge protest.
- In Europe, they launched an advertising campaign attempting to promote the use of genetically engineered crops and this has led to African scientists expressing their concern as well.
- They are also accused of creating products that will withstand more pesticide use and therefore allow more sales of their pesticide products. (Note, as mentioned above, they are largely a chemical and pesticide company.) Genetically engineered for

Roundup Ready Soybeans, for example, are engineered to be more resistant to its Roundup weed killer. That weed killer also kills many beneficial "weeds" and insects. This doesn't have much to do with increasing yields as studies have shown but more about increased sales.

A quote says it all:

"Many of you have heard of Monsanto's Roundup herbicide. In addition, it's very effective at killing weeds -- so effective, in fact, that Roundup would control soybeans as well as weeds if it should come into contact as both. ... [Until that is,] Monsanto developed Roundup Ready Soybeans ... [that] express a novel protein that allows them to survive, even when sprayed with enough Roundup to control competing weeds."

- — from the International Association of Plant Breeders, quoted by Vanadana Shiva, Stolen Harvest (South End Press, 2000), p.98 Also, see Vanadana Shiva, Stolen Harvest (South End Press, 2000), pp.99 - 101 for more about the "Myth of Increased Yields and Returns".

An example of corporate control and propaganda Monsanto has on issues, on April 2, 1998, two award-winning Florida TV producers announced a lawsuit against a Fox TV network television station, which they claim, had fired them after they refused to broadcast false reports about Monsanto's controversial genetically engineered <u>Bovine Growth Hormone</u>. This hormone is said to harm cows and pose risks to humans. Due to public pressure, Canada, for example, has refused to allow it to be used.

The Ecologists publication in the UK bowed to pressure from the Company and destroyed an article on this for fear of being sued. In addition, in the UK, it has been shown that a Monsanto Lobby firm is paying a key member of parliament thousands of pounds. The MP is in charge of the influential House of Commons committee policing Government food policy. There are similar charges of a "revolving door" at the USA's Food and Drug Administration (FDA) where former Monsanto employees end up at the FDA and back to Monsanto again.

Basically, the Company has managed to buy its way into the very system designed to protect the public making going after them nearly impossible.

It is not just Monsanto that has come under fire for its policies. Virtually all of the chemical Industry has similar problems and a similar influence over farming and the FDA itself. As an example, in September 2000, there was a fiasco in the United States about genetically modified taco shells in the food system using genetically engineered corn that was not approved for human consumption. It highlighted a series of concerns about gene spills, and, also less mentioned and analyzed by the US press, the corporate policies of accountability and general lack of such. On the manufacturing side in the Beef industry, we just had the whole Pink Slime issue a few months back.

The full report on the Taco issue is as follows:

"In studying [the taco] case we are struck by the dense network of transnational corporations (TNCs) involved, and the relationships between them -- symptomatic, we feel, of larger problems in our food system. A food processor (Kraft) owned by a tobacco company (Phillip Morris), pays a licensing fee to the world's largest fast food corporation (Tricon, which owns Taco Bell, KFC, and Pizza Hut), itself a spin-off from PepsiCo, and buys the taco shells from a direct subsidiary of Pepsi (Sabritas), who bought the flour from the company (Gruma) who produces over half of the tortillas consumed in the world and is partially owned by the nation's largest grain processor (ADM), a major campaign contributor to both political parties, found guilty at various times of price fixing and anti-trust violations. ADM in turn bought the corn from farmers who bought the seed from a biotech conglomerate (Aventis Crop Science), formed by the merger of two chemical companies (AgrEvo and Rhône-Poulenc), one of whom (AgrEvo) is itself the product of the previous merger of the Hoechst and Schering pharmaceutical and pesticide giants. Where does the buck stop? Who is to blame? If GE Food Alert hadn't paid for independent testing, who would have?

... As fewer companies come to dominate each step in food

production, whether supplying farmers with seeds and chemicals, processing food, or retailing through supermarkets, there are fewer checks and balances in the system.

When an industry is competitive -- when there are many companies producing similar products, each with a small market share -- consumers have a better shot at getting what they need and want, and government regulators are less likely to be in the pockets of giant conglomerates. However, when oligopolies or monopolies achieve preeminent positions in the market, they can unilaterally raise prices and cut costs, allowing quality to deteriorate because consumers are captive-they have no choice. In addition, the windfall profits that accrue to dominant market positions make it possible-and necessary to protect those profits-to influence regulators through the revolving door between government and industry, campaign contributions and outright payoffs.

Since it is the transnational corporations which are the beneficiaries of the long history of inequity that has plagued us in our position of disadvantage, I believe that it is our responsibility to reject such a misleading oversimplification of the solution to our problem; especially the use of our condition, by those very beneficiaries of the inequity, to justify the continuation of the benefits that they derive."

— Anatomy of a 'Gene Spill', Institute for Food and Development Policy (Food First)

Further,:

"Farmers in the U.S. have already have had non-GMO crops contaminated by nearby GMO fields. Currently farmers have no recourse in such situations, since there is no legal protection from this bio-pollution. Farmers who lose premiums for their non-GMO or organic crop have nowhere to turn. Biotech industry spokespeople have suggested that farmers who are concerned about such contamination should take part of their land out of production as "buffer zones." Obviously farmers who are doing nothing different than before feel that they should not now be burdened by the industry's failure to control its technology."

— Bill Christison, <u>Opposing Genetic Engineering In New Zealand (and around the world)</u>, In Motion Magazine, February 25, 2001

Monsanto is a biotechnology firm. They are genetically manipulating seed to perform as they wish and they have gone into federal patent courts and had the patents granted. Now they own the patent on their Roundup Ready seeds, as they call them. Essentially, they developed a seed that was resistant to Round up weed killer, so you could weed your field without killing your product. Well, that sounds like a good thing, what's wrong with that? Nothing if that were all there was to the problem. However, it was Monsanto's ability to claim a field was their seed, if seed was never planted in the field. The idea that cross-pollination can takes place when the wind blows, or a truck transporting the product passes by and blows it into your field, or any other of the different ways a field becomes cross pollinated. When Monsanto sued Mr. Schmeiser, a farmer who kept his own seed because of evidence such had taken place, in the federal courts of Canada the judge, one Mr. Andrew McKay upheld the patent of Monsanto's that a field of product that had become cross pollinated by no means of the farmer who owns the land, became the property of the of the patent owner because of the genetically modified seed is owned by Monsanto. Generally Canadian law protects a farmer from cross-pollination claims due to mother nature, but not for genetically modified plants. Mother Nature no longer owns those plants, the modifier does.

What the Company has done is literally become able to claim almost any seed out there under these same grounds. In effect, they almost have begun to own nature, and not nature owns them. No matter if you are an evolutionist, religionist or just plain consumer of food, this is wrong. Plant life and animal life springs forth on its own, without help from human beings. The act of genetically modifying them to produce superior results is wrong. We are going in the wrong direction when we allow a corporation to manipulate the food we eat in a laboratory with nothing short of a lifetime of testing or at least follow up testing that would be required for any other product out there in the World. There is also the need to limit their ability to claim a Farmers harvest just because of the whole cross-pollination, which by the way, generally takes place under natural events like wind, etc.

As Forbes has pointed out on their website,

"Monsanto, the world's largest agriculture seed producer, is under fire after scientists in the U.S. recently discovered what they believe to be a case of crop-eating bugs developing a resistance to the company's genetically modified corn plants. Some researchers believe that the discovery validates concerns that biotech crops could spawn new species of pesticide-resistant super-bugs. Among Environmental, Social, Governance (ESG) circles, reports of this phenomenon have sparked discussions about the importance of corporate social responsibility (CSR) policies when it comes to environmental issues."

This is another whole issue out there little studied and could in itself pose a major threat to the World food supply. The problem is these Companies will not regulate themselves because it weakens their bottom line. Only regulation at a Government level and forced testing of products will change this situation, not deregulation which tends to promote more of what we already have in this Industry far too much of.

Monsanto has faced criticism for marketing products that have the potential to cause serious environmental damage many times in the past. They have a long history of caring little about public safety in general. For two decades, Monsanto has produced and marketed seeds that can survive exposure to the company's Roundup herbicide, a powerful chemical with a strong reputation for being an effective weed-killer.

The problem is, these Roundup resistant seeds made it easy for farmers to plant crops and then douse them with Monsanto pesticide, that many farms abandoned other techniques. Now, according to a number of scientific reports, super weeds that are immune to Monsanto's pesticides have spread to millions of acres in more than 20 states the Midwestern United States. In general, one has to ask if the real Business of this Company is nothing more than profit at the expense of the health and welfare of everyone else in the world.

They are kind of like those Generals in the War Pigs song who bow before God in the end begging mercy for having destroyed the world. The actual better question is do they know all this ahead of time and have plans on new products to go after these super bugs and super weeds given their general foreknowledge in the past in cases like Agent Orange? Then the question becomes what if one day all this leads to weeds and bugs nothing can stop? Who do they bow down to and beg forgiveness when that happens?

As Bill Freese, a science policy analyst for the Center for Food Safety in Washington explained that "the biotech industry is taking us into a more pesticide-dependent agriculture… we need to be going in, the opposite direction."

However, Companies like this are full speed ahead with the turbo at full in the direction of more and more stronger chemicals in our fields and eventually in our food supply chain while the FDA gets controlled by them, and no one is forced to find out the long term effects such has on the Consumer.

In 2011 Monsanto was fined by the U.S. Environmental Protection Agency for contaminating water supplies near one of its rural U.S. facilities and targeted for investigation by the U.S. Securities and Exchange Commission for making cash incentive payments to farmers who use its herbicides. Monsanto is becoming a fertile ground for discussion of corporate environmental policies and responsibilities, however, almost no one is forcing this discussion at a level that can change anything of their current policy. The FDA will not do it because they are in bed with Companies like this to begin with. The Senate, especially GOP controlled ones, will do everything to not further regulate companies like this. So, who besides us the Consumer via what we buy can do anything to control all this? Money talks, and Bull Shit walks, is an old saying. Our money can dictate change in the whole Farming Industry simply via altering what we buy at the market. If it is not Organic, do not buy it is the simplest way to force Companies like this to self regulate or go out of business.

More than 800 million pounds of pesticides are used on agriculture crops in this country each year. This amounts to about four pounds for each person in the United States. Despite these large volumes being applied to the nation's food supply, studies show that pesticide residues are "nearly always well below" legal limits. However, there is a catch in all this. All the testing assumes what is a safe single dose of these in our food. Nowhere do they actually look at long-term effects of multiple doses over the life of any individual. The (EPA) approves and registers the use of pesticides applied to food products in the field. After a legal residue level has been established for a pesticide, the U.S. Department of Agriculture (USDA) and the FDA are responsible for ensuring that limits are not exceeded. However, as we have already encountered the FDA is mostly manned by retired members of Companies like Monsanto to begin with and might as well be controlled by them. So who holds the FDA to account considering they are part of the Government to begin with that has proven over and over again it cannot be trusted?

The EPA has approved legal limits for approximately 300 Pesticides. Pesticides are chemicals used to eliminate or control a variety of agricultural pests that can damage crops and livestock and reduce farm productivity. The most commonly applied pesticides are insecticides (to kill insects), herbicides (to kill weeds), rodenticides (to kill rodents), and fungicides (to control fungi, mold, and mildew). Of these pesticide classes, herbicides (weed killers) are the most widely used, with Round Up being the number on out there. Today, approximately 5.1 billion pounds of pesticides are used in the US every year.

Approximately 37% of the world's grain and 66% of U.S. grain is used for livestock feed. This grain is grown by intensive farming operations that use massive quantities of pesticides while producing problems such as pesticide resistance in insects and weeds, and pollution of nearby water supplies with toxic chemicals. It also makes it into the meat we eat via what the livestock consumes that was treated with these agents. Many grain crops are genetic modified, so that the plants are bred either to contain pesticides within their entire genetic makeup or to withstand direct application of chemical pesticides or herbicides. Furthermore, when grain is grown with pesticides and then fed to livestock, pesticide residues accumulate in the animals' fatty tissue. Here again, no long term study of this accumulated effect on the animals or on us. The best example of the Scientific Community looking at this and sounding a alarm comes via:

Walker, Polly, et al. "Public Health Implications of Meat Production and

Consumption," Invited Paper, Public Health Nutrition: 8(4), 348-356. Johns Hopkins University, 2005.

However, this is just one voice sounding an alarm with many more remaining silent on the issue for fear of being bullied by the chemical companies.

Further,:

A 2004 analysis of Centers for Disease Control (CDC) data revealed that 100% of blood and urine tests from subjects they monitored showed pesticide residues. Two insecticides — chlorpyrifos and methyl parathion — were found at levels up to 4.6 times greater than what the US government deems acceptable.
Schafer S., Kristin, et al. "Chemical Trespass: Pesticides in Our Bodies and Corporate Accountability." Pesticide Action Network of North America, May 2004.

In a joint study conducted by scientists from the CDC, the University of Washington and Emory University, researchers found that pesticide levels in test subjects dropped to undetectable levels upon switching to an organic diet. When the subjects switched back to a non-organic diet, pesticide residues almost immediately became detectable.
Lu, Chenseng, Kathryn Toepel, Rene Irish, Richard A. Fenske, Dana B. Barr, Roberto Bravo, "Organic Diets Significantly Lower Children's Dietary Exposure to Organophosphorus Pesticides." Environmental Health Perspectives, Volume 114, Number 2, February 2006.

According to Cornell entomologist David Pimentel, "It has been estimated that only 0.1% of applied pesticides reach the target pests, leaving the bulk of the pesticides (99.9%) to impact the environment. Basically, they eventually also make it into our water supply.

Pesticides are a health concern and have been linked to a range of diseases and disorders. Many chemical pesticides are known to cause poisoning, infertility and birth defects, as well as damage the nervous system and potentially cause cancer. Research has shown that many people in the US carry high levels of pesticides in their bodies. This comes from a lot of origin points including that run off into the water supply.

Pesticide Action Network of North America. "Toxic Pesticides Above "Safe" Levels in Many U.S.Residents." May 2004.

The EPA's methods for testing pesticides are insufficient because they only examine the effects of exposure to pesticides at high doses. Without conducting research concerning long-term exposure to low doses of pesticides, these studies neglect to base safety levels on real-life situations. Moreover, the tests examine the effects of a single chemical, whereas people are typically contaminated with small amounts of hundreds of pesticides at any one time due to the fact that we do not just consume one type of food or all drink water outside of our public supply.

The FDA is inadequate in monitoring of pesticide levels on fruits and vegetables. The Environmental Working Group reports that the FDA fails to test the majority of produce consumed in the US, and as a result Americans regularly consume food-bearing residues of illegal pesticides that are not approved for use in the US because we now have food coming to our stores from Mexico and other Countries with no FDA regulation of any kind.

Environmental Working Group, "Why reducing pesticide exposure is smart." EWG, 2005.

In some cases when a pesticide is known to have harmful breakdown products, a tolerance limit may be set for the total amount of "parent" pesticide and breakdown products that may be present in or on food. In such cases, foods may be tested for all these residues. For example, tolerances have been established for the total amount of the pesticide endosulfan and its breakdown product endosulfan sulfate. However, here again, this is all based upon averages that no where take into account long term exposure to such, and in this case, only look at the break down within the food itself, not the human body. For example, the pesticides triclopyr, chlorpyrifos and chlorpyrifos-methyl all release the breakdown product, 3,5,6-trichloro-2-pyridinol (TCP) a known health problem.

From the survey in 1997, FDA reported volatile residues in domestic foods in 16 of 1,171 (1.2%) fruits and 41 of 1,707 (2.4%) vegetables. No volatile residues were found in milk, dairy products, eggs, bananas, apple juice, grains and grain products, and seafood, even though sea food has a mercury problem. Among the imported food samples, 3 of 322 (0.9%) grain and grain products, 24 of 2,034 (1.2%) fruits, 50 of 2,356 (2.1%) vegetables, and 7 of 268 (2.6%) samples of other products such as nuts and spices had volatile residues. No volatile residues were found in imported milk, dairy products, eggs, seafood, bananas and apple juice.

Besides monitoring pesticide residues in raw agricultural produce before it reaches the market, the FDA also conducts "Total Diet Studies." The USDA's Nationwide Food Consumption Surveys provide information on what people eat or what is a "typical meal." Total Diet Studies are designed to determine pesticide residues in commonly eaten menu items such as macaroni and cheese, chicken nuggets, pop corn and ice cream. The three most common residues found in such studies were the insecticides DDT, malathion and chlorpyrifos-methyl. These residues were not above the acceptable or tolerance limits. However, no long term build up study has ever been done.

The next problem in our food supply involves growth hormones. The use of growth hormones in food production processes is a regular practice within the meat and dairy industries. Producers depend on these chemicals to achieve larger livestock, better quality meats and increased dairy production levels. The Food and Drug Administration is responsible for monitoring the safety of the foods we eat. But, here again, we run into the problem of Big Corporations buying off the Government designed to do such monitoring, and in many cases, like with Monsanto, people from those same companies working within the FDA.

With the case of milk production, a synthetic chemical called rb GH, also known as bovine growth hormone, is injected into cows to increase the length of their lactation periods. With meat, as many as six different hormones are used within the production process.

Zeronal, trenbolone and melengestrol are synthetics used to promote growth in livestock, whereas, oestradiol, progesterone and testosterone are naturally-based. Melengestol is also used as a feed additive. All those in use actually are synthetic hormones.

Certain synthetic hormones used to treat humans were found to increase the risk of cancers. Diethylstilbestrol (DES), a synthetic estrogen, was used in the1960s to reduce the risk of miscarriage for women. It was eventually banned as a result of research studies that found a link between DES and vaginal cancer in the offspring of women who had been treated with the drug. This, and other accounts have raised considerable concern as to what effects the growth hormones in our food can have. Studies carried out on rats by Health Canada (Canada's version of our FDA) were given the rb GH synthetic used for milk production in cows. Results showed the rats systems' had built up anti-bodies to milk as result of rb GH. These results seem to indicate that synthetic hormones can give rise to milk allergies, or lactose intolerance in humans. There is also the bigger question of how well this drugs designed to speed up growth are impacting our youth which, current studies have indicated, are maturing, body wise, at a far younger age than in the past.

As early as the 1930s, it was realized that cows injected with material drawn from bovine (cow) pituitary glands (hormone secreting organ) produced more milk. Later, the bovine growth hormone (bGH) from the pituitary glands was found to be responsible for this effect. However, at that time, technology did not exist to harvest enough of this material for large-scale use in animals. In the 1980s, it became possible to produce large quantities of pure bGH by using recombinant DNA technology. In 1993, the Food and Drug Administration (FDA) approved the recombinant bovine growth hormone (rbGH), also known as bovine somatotropin (rbST) for use in dairy cattle. Recent estimates by the manufacturer of this hormone indicate that 30% of the cows in the United States (US) may be treated with rbGH.

The female sex hormone estrogen was also shown to affect growth rates in cattle and poultry in the 1930s. Once the chemistry of estrogen was understood, it became possible to make the hormone synthetically in large amounts. Synthetic estrogens started being used to increase the size of cattle and chickens in the early 1950s. DES was one of the first synthetic estrogens made and used commercially in the US to fatten chickens. DES was also used as a drug in human medicine. DES was found to cause cancer and its use in food production was phased out in the late 1970s.

Early puberty in girls has been found to be associated with a higher risk for breast cancer. Height, weight, diet, exercise, and family history have all been found to influence age of puberty. Steroid hormones in food were suspected to cause early puberty in girls in some reports. Large epidemiological studies have not been done to see whether or not early puberty in developing girls is associated with having eaten growth hormone-treated foods. Basically, though we have tracking medical evidence that shows our children are aging quicker, both boys and girls, over the time period such hormones have been being used, no lab to date has ever done a long term study on this subject. What this amounts to is a smoking gun signature, without a valid study to prove the smoking gun exists.

In 1989, the European Community (now European Union) issued a ban on all meat from animals treated with steroid growth hormones, which is still in effect. The use of steroid hormones for beef cattle is permitted in Canada.

Countries within the European Union do not allow the use of the protein hormone rbGH, for dairy cattle. In 1999, the Canadian government refused approval for the sale of rbGH for dairy cattle, based on concerns about the health effects including mastitis in treated animals. However, in this Country to date no such bans exist and we continue to ingest food with these hormones in them.

According to the European Union's Scientific Committee on Veterinary Measures Relating to Public Health, the use of six natural and artificial growth hormones in beef production poses a potential risk to human health. These six hormones include three which are naturally occurring—Oestradiol, Progesterone and Testosterone—and three which are synthetic—Zeranol, Trenbolone, and Melengestrol.

The Committee also questioned whether hormone residues in the meat of "growth enhanced" animals and can disrupt human hormone balance, causing developmental problems, interfering with the reproductive system, and even leading to the development of breast, prostate or colon cancer.

Growth promoting hormones remain in the meat we consume, but they also pass through the cattle and are excreted in their manure. When manure from factory farms enters the surrounding environment, these hormones can contaminate surface and groundwater. Aquatic ecosystems are particularly vulnerable to hormone residues. Recent studies have demonstrated that exposure to hormones has a substantial effect on the gender and reproductive capacity of fish, throwing off the natural cycle.

FDA approval for rBGH came in 1993, in spite of strong opposition from scientists, farmers and consumers. According to detractors, rBGH was never properly tested. The FDA relied solely on a study done by Monsanto in which rBGH was tested for 90 days on 30 rats. The study was never published, and the FDA stated the results showed no significant problems. But a review by the Canadian health agency on rBGH found the 90 day study showed a significant number of issues which should have triggered a full review by the FDA. Again we have Monsanto and the FDA in bed together, since they are the leading chemical company involved in the food industry.

By the summer of 1994, the Wisconsin Farmers Union and the National Farmers Union set up a joint hotline for dairy farmers to use when reporting problems with the artificial growth hormones in cattle. One lifelong New York dairy farmer reported losing a quarter of his herd to severe mastitis after beginning rBGH injections. He also reported a drastic drop in production after taking his cows off rBGH; they suddenly produced less milk then they had before going on the drug. A year later, he had to replace 135 of his original 200 cows. Other farmers using rBGH have reported similar problems, in addition to hoof diseases, open sores and cows that died from internal bleeding.

A 1991 report by Vermont revealed serious health problems with the rBGH-injected cows that were part of a Monsanto-financed study at the University of Vermont (UVM). Among the problems was an alarming rise in the number of deformed calves and dramatic increases in mastitis, a painful bacterial infection of the udder which causes inflammation and swelling. To treat mastitis outbreaks, the dairy industry has relied on antibiotics. Critics of rBGH point to the subsequent increase in antibiotic use, which contributes to the growing problem of antibiotic resistant bacteria, and, inadequacies in the federal government's testing program for antibiotic residues in milk. Basically, not only was Monsanto involved in this case, they had the evidence right there in one of their own study groups and simply addressed the issue with another chemical band-aid being added into our food supply.

Milk from rBGH-treated cows contains higher levels of IGF-1 (Insulin Growth Factor-1), which has been linked to colon and breast cancer. Even though no direct connection has been made between elevated IGF-1 levels in milk and cancer in humans, scientists have expressed concern.

See:

Raloff, Janet. "Hormones: Here's the Beef: environmental concerns reemerge over steroids given to livestock." Science News 161, no. 1, January 5, 2002, 10.
Kastel, Mark, "Down on the Farm: The Real BGH Story Animal Health Problems, Financial Troubles." Rural Vermont, 1995.
Hansen, Michael, Jean M. Halloran, Edward Groth III, and Lisa Y. Lefferts, Potential Public Health Impacts Of The Use Of Recombinant Bovine Somatotropin In Dairy Production: Prepared for a Scientific Review by the Joint Expert Committee on Food Additives, September 1997.
Schneider, Keith, "F.D.A. Warns the Dairy Industry Not to Label Milk Hormone-Free," New York Times, February 8, 1994.
Schiffer, Bettina, Andreas Daxenberger, Karsten Meyer, and Heinrich H.D. Meyer. " The Fate of Trenbolone Acetate and Melengestrol Acetate after Application as Growth Promoters in Cattle: Environmental Studies." Environmental Health Perspectives. 109, no. 11, November 2001, 1145.

According to Science News, 80 percent of all U.S. feedlot cattle are injected with hormones. A study of cows treated with melengestrol acetate (one of the artificial growth hormones approved for use in the U.S.) revealed that residues of this hormone were traceable in soil up to 195 days after being administered to the animals. While the average dairy cow produced almost 5,300 pounds of milk a year in 1950, today, a typical cow produces more than 18,000 pounds.

Faced with mounting evidence to the contrary, the FDA has stubbornly continued to assure consumers that rBGH and other hormones are safe for cows and humans.   However, when you follow the money trail from Monsanto to the Government, and look at the individuals coming out of Monsanto into the FDA it is easy to see why this remains this way.   Basically, the FDA has become a puppet of Monsanto and other giant companies like it, with you and I, the consumers, becoming the lab rats when it comes to our food supply.   The simplest solution is cut out the middle man, the FDA, by buying organic grown food in the first place and avoiding any chance the FDA really does care about us. You cut the bottom line out of Monsanto and you prevent your health having to depend upon an FDA already shown to be negligent in their duty to protect the American People.

If you think fish is a safe bet, a genetically engineered salmon patented by the biotech company AquaBounty. If the salmon, which is wired to produce growth hormone year-round, instead of just in the spring and summer, gets an OK from the FDA, it will be the first genetically engineered animal to wind up on your dinner plate. Genetically engineered fruits and vegetables have been around for years, which might have gone unnoticed by some.

A three-ounce serving of beef from an estrogen-treated cow contains less than a billionth of a gram of estrogen, a level around 400,000 times lower than estrogen in women and nearly 100,000 times lower than that in men.   However, no study of long term build up has ever been done, neither has the fact that on an average most American's consume far more than three ounces of beef in a day.   In fact, this is well below the average offering on a burger or a steak on a menu in this country. A 2009 study found that children who consumed the most protein from animal sources entered puberty about seven months earlier than those who consumed the least.   Again, the FDA, in bed with Monsanto continues to ignore all these studies.

These hormones survive digestion and are readily absorbed from the small intestine into the blood. Increased levels of IGF-1 have been shown to increase risks of breast cancer in 19 scientific publications, risks of colon cancer in 10 publications, and prostate cancer in seven publications. Of further concern, increased IGF-1 levels block natural defense mechanisms against early microscopic cancers, known as apoptosis. The Cancer Prevention Coalition, endorsed by five leading national experts, petitioned the FDA in May 2007 to label rBGH milk with an explicit cancer warnings. In the absence of any response, they resubmitted this petition in January 2010 to Dr. Hamburg, and are waiting for a response. Basically, they are waiting on Monsanto to indorse those labels which stands a snow balls chance in hell of being done.

Again, the simplest solution that gets around this whole illicit Monsanto/FDA love affair is to buy organic and avoid the problem to begin with. The FDA, besides the USDA, have failed to take any regulatory action to protect the public from the dangers of hormonal meat. A 1986 report, "Human Food Safety and Regulation of Animal Drugs," unanimously approved by the House Committee on Government Operations, concluded that the "FDA has consistently disregarded its responsibility, has repeatedly put what it perceives are interests of veterinarians and the livestock industry ahead of its legal obligation to protect consumers, jeopardizing the health and safety of consumers meat, milk, and poultry." And the reason both of these Government agencies have failed to do so all goes back to the control and influence companies like Monsanto have over them both within those agencies and in Congress.

Again, the solution is plain: Cut the money tree off at the root for Companies like Monsanto. If you buy organic there is currently no profit in it for Monsanto. Cut their money off by not buying the food doctored with their chemicals and they cease to have any power over anything to do with our food supply. You simply force via how and what you consume the rest of the Farmers out there to quit using Monsanto products and take back control of your health for yourself without having to rely upon any Government Agency known to be not trust worthy.

The Drug Industry

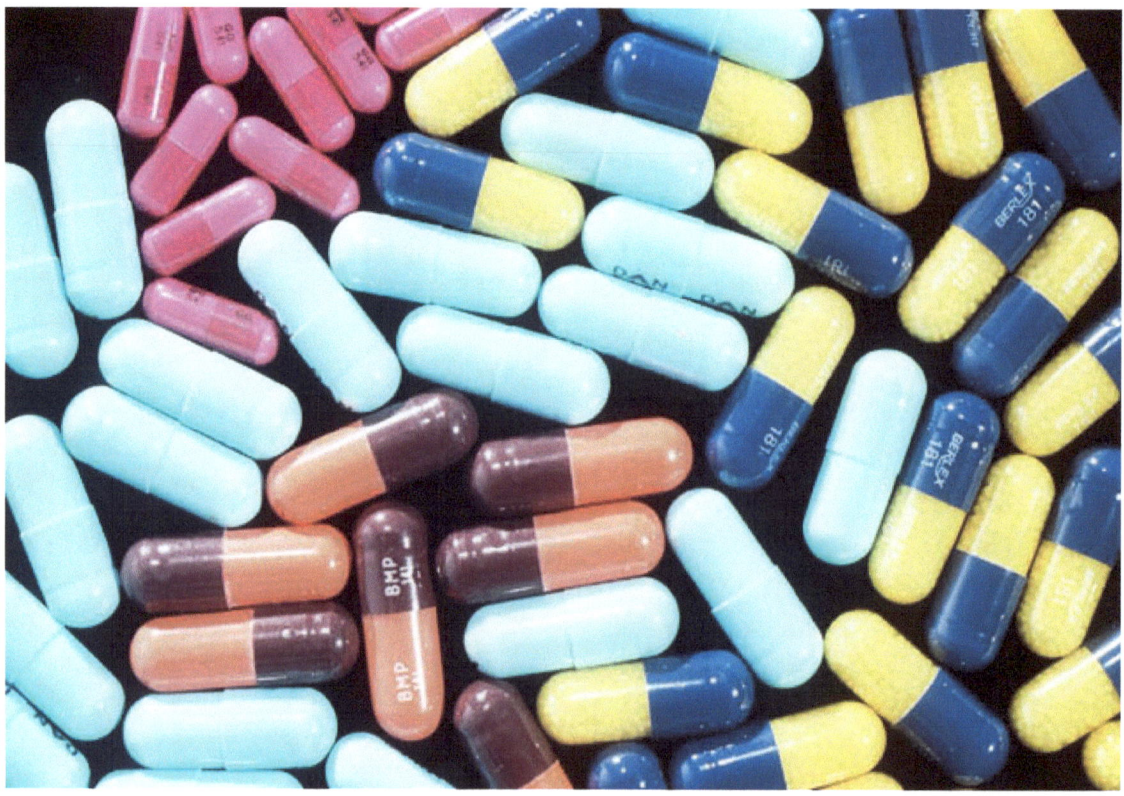

Crime pays. As just two recent examples, Pfizer was fined a record $2.3 Billion in September 2009, which represents less than three weeks of sales for the company); and in January 2009, Eli Lilly was fined $1.4 Billion. Drugs like Vioxx (made by Merck) are profitable such that the drug companies see people getting killed and criminal fines as mere costs of doing business. Put simple, the drug Companies do not care about the people who use their drugs. They only care about their bottom line. Who is supposed to watch over all this and protect us? You got it. The FDA, same FDA in bed over money on our food problem is same agency in bed with another sort of chemical company group, the drug manufacture.

More than 50% of the people who advise the FDA on drug safety have a financial interest in the decision. Although federal law says that this is illegal, exceptions are granted regularly. As just one example, between January 1998 and June 2000, the FDA granted 800 waivers to the rule. Roughly 100,000 people a year die from OTC (over the counter) and prescription drugs. The only other worse culprits are: cancer, heart disease and stroke. In the last 25 years, 20 percent of the approved drugs have either been recalled (ie. Vioxx) or have had new labels added warning of extreme side effects. Sidney Taurel, chairman of Eli Lilly, admits "The typical Food and Drug Administration approved drug is effective on just 50 percent of patients."

They promote "disease management" over true preventative health care. Most of the drugs on the market today only

1) cover up the true issue;

2) create addictions;

3) have side effects that are worse than what's being treated;

4) actually cause the condition to get worse than before.

Simply put, healthy people don't create profits. The drug industry gets the highest profit margins from creating "lifetime users". There is no honest profit in any cure at all.

Drug companies create the drug, then they pay for the clinical research used to study its' safety and effectiveness. The public and physicians are led to believe that impartial research institutions are conducting the studies. The little known truth is that today, over 90% of safety and effectiveness research is financed directly by the drug companies. The drug manufacturers carefully stack the decks in their favor, throw away studies that don't show the desired outcomes and put researchers under pressure to "get the right results." Basically, they side step any real honest testing and peer review all in the name of the bottom line leaving us, the consumer of these pills again as Lab Rats all because the FDA is bought and sold by the highest bidder.

There is strong evidence that associations between industry and doctors influence the behaviour of the latter in relation to both clinical decision making and the conduct of research. In 2009 alone, the number of serious problems and deaths linked to medications reported to the government set a record in the first three months of that year. Fresh in 2012's headlines is the whole affair with the New England Compounding Company, again ignored for the most part by the FDA, who instead of leveling a few years back heavy fines, due to similar problems, basically slapped them on the wrist because the Company in response had said it would cause an undue burden.

The Food and Drug Administration received nearly 21,000 reports of serious drug reactions, including over 4,800 deaths, said an analysis of federal data by the nonprofit Institute for Safe Medication Practices, which scrutinized data going back to 2004, and yearly totals dating to the 1990s. Two drugs stood out. They where heparin, the tainted blood thinner from China that caused an international safety scandal. The other was Chantix, a new kind of anti-smoking drug from Pfizer.

The FDA defines serious drug reactions as ones that cause hospitalization, require medical intervention, or place a life in jeopardy. The agency's monitoring system relies on voluntary reports from doctors and is only believed to capture a fraction of overall problems. Basically, they only step in when something goes wrong, like in the case of NECC, not all along as they should. The agency split by fierce disagreements that have not been resolved by repeated reorganizations and management efforts. Indeed, managers' failure to address such disagreements competently has played an important role in damaging the credibility of the F.D.A.. This has been born out by almost every independent agency looking at the FDA for years now. They are under staffed, to easily bought off, too often lax on their own duties, and almost never catch problems before they surface in the public.

The Institute of Medicine(IOM), panel made important recommendations that would put the agency back on track to fulfill its mission of protecting the public health instead of industry's cash flow:

Put a symbol on the packages of new drugs to denote that the medicine's benefits and risks may not be fully understood. It would remain in pace for two years.

Ban advertising directed at patients during that two-year period.

Review the risks and benefits of all new drugs after five years.

Bolster the Food and Drug Administration's safety staff and give it an integral role in drug approval.

Give FDA legal authority to order drug companies to conduct safety studies and to institute other precautions to protect patients.

Modernize and extend the FDA's databases for tracking serious reactions to prescription drugs.

Create an Internet registry to post results of clinical drug trials.

Adopt stronger policies to minimize conflicts of interest among outside advisors who serve on the panels that guide much of the FDA's work.

Establish a six-year term for the FDA commissioner, who now serves at the pleasure of the president, to provide stable leadership.

At the current time, the Food and Drug Administration must negotiate safety warning labels with a drug maker when in reality, if a drug is known to have problem such a label should be a requirement to continue sales of the drug. Pharmaceutical companies should disclose the results of ALL clinical trials, not just the ones with positive results that they wish to publicize. Currently, drug companies can bury negative drug trials, and the FDA has in fact been caught conspiring with drug companies to keep negative drug data secret from the public. Currently, the FDA has no authority to require follow-up safety studies on drugs after they are introduced to the market. This is a serious shortfall in oversight, given that many problems with drugs only appear after widespread use, like in the NECC case and many others.

At the current time doctors and scientists with a financial conflict of interest are allowed to serve on FDA advisory board. Basically, the one's who stand to make money on these drugs are the one dictating the FDA. Sounds no different than what goes on in the Food Industry.

According to the Journal of the American Medical Association, prescription drugs currently kill approximately 100,000 Americans each year. However, very few of these cases ever come across the FDA desk or even get mentioned to Congress.

The makers of Vioxx and Paxil had studies that indicated safety problems for years, but did not release those results to the public. The NECC, had a long list of problems going back years, including a law suit over a death in 03 for same situation paid off out of court all documented by the FDA in their own records and nothing was done resulting in multiple deaths and sick people across the Country. What is worse, the people who worked at this Company knew of an on going problem and stood by and did nothing. All of this under the so called watchful eye of our Government, who got paid off to look the other way.

The real question not being asked is how many Americans do you think is acceptable for the drug companies to kill each year? That same question needs brought up before Congress who is supposed to have over sight over the FDA. Problem is, if you are waiting on that one to be asked you are backing up, especially with our current politically divided do nothing Congress that cannot even come together to pass a budget. This lame brain, over paid couch potato Congress would never act unless perhaps someone in their family died.

Dr. Marcia Angell argues that problems with the industry run even deeper. In her new book, The Truth About Drug Companies: How They Deceive Us and What to Do About It , the former editor of the New England Journal of Medicine contends that the industry has become a marketing machine that produces few innovative drugs and is dependent on monopoly rights and public-sponsored research. Not unlike the problem with the Chemical Companies and the Food Industry and their control on the FDA. Angell disputes the industry's reputation as an "engine of innovation," arguing that the top U.S. drug makers spend 2.5 times as much on marketing and administration as they do on research. At least a third of the drugs marketed by industry leaders were discovered by universities or small biotech companies, writes Angell, but they're sold to the public at inflated prices.

All of this stands as proof over and over again that their bottom line, not our safety is priority. And it is that bottom line that drives and dictates the FDA over and over again. The FDA has become an agency in dire need of a fire sale. From the Top on down a message needs to be sent that we require them to do the job they where created and paid to do or get out so we can find some who will. The place to start that fire sale is with Congress. They are the one's who need to get the message that the American People have had enough. And the Fire Sale needs to be across Party lines considering both sides are guilty of allowing this to go on.

Conclusions:

The simplest way to deal with our food supply problems is alter how and what we buy at the Markets. Put Companies like Monsanto out of business when it comes to our food supply. The simplest way to deal with the problem in our drugs is start a fire sale and letter campaign to those in Congress. Alter the do nothing mind set in Washington and you can change the FDA for the better.